HOW FAST CAN I LOSE WEIGHT

RAPID WEIGHT LOSS STRATEGIES FOR ALL

A.D RAMS

Contents

CHAPTER ONE

INTRODUCTION

When starting a weight loss journey, "How fast can I lose weight?" is a common question asked by many. It makes sense to want rapid results, but it's important to approach weight loss with a sustainable and realistic perspective. While drastic workout plans or crash diets may be effective in the short term, they frequently result in long-term health hazards and rebound weight gain. Long-term success can instead be achieved by concentrating on small, sustainable improvements to your food, exercise routine, and way of life. We'll look at what affects weight loss pace in this guide, along with methods for reaching healthy, long-term weight loss and advice on how to create reasonable goals for yourself on the path to better health.

addressing the need to lose weight quickly

The urge for speedy results is common in today's fast-paced environment, and weight loss is no exception. Many people look for quick weight loss methods in an effort to reach their objectives as soon as feasible. Although it makes sense to want results right away, it's crucial to be aware of the hazards and restrictions connected to quick weight reduction methods.

Health concerns: There are a number of serious health concerns associated with rapid weight loss techniques including crash diets and severe calorie restriction. These methods frequently lack vital nutrients, which can result in immune system weakness, exhaustion, muscle loss, and nutritional shortages. Rapid weight reduction may also raise the risk of electrolyte imbalances, gallstones, and other health issues.

Muscle Loss: Along with fat loss, rapid weight loss, mostly due to calorie restriction, can also cause muscle loss. Long-term weight maintenance may be more difficult as a result of this, as it may have a detrimental effect on metabolism and body composition. Maintaining muscle mass is critical for general strength and function, as well as a healthy metabolism.

Metabolic Adaptation: Crash diets and excessive calorie restriction might cause metabolic changes that impede attempts to lose weight. It may be more difficult to lose weight when the body slows down metabolism to conserve energy when it isn't getting enough calories. Weight gain may result from this metabolic adaption, which may last even after one returns to regular eating habits.

Nutritional Imbalance: Quick weight loss techniques frequently ignore nutritional balance in favor of cutting calories alone. This may lead to insufficient consumption of vital nutrients, which are critical for general health and wellbeing and include vitamins, minerals, and protein. Inadequate nutrition can lead to various health problems and have long-term effects on health.

Sustainability: Although rapid weight loss can produce immediate results, it is frequently not long-term sustainable. Extreme workout routines and crash diets are hard to stick to over time and can cause feelings of deprivation, anger, and fatigue. A sustainable weight loss plan calls for incremental, long-term adjustments to your lifestyle, nutrition, and level of physical activity.

Psychological Impact: Trying to lose weight quickly might be detrimental to one's mental and emotional health. If weight loss goals are not rapidly achieved, pursuing fast fixes and having irrational expectations can result in feelings of failure, guilt, and humiliation. Prioritizing mental health and implementing a well-rounded weight-loss strategy that encourages self-care and self-compassion are crucial.

Though it's normal to want to lose weight quickly, it's crucial to approach weight loss from a sustainable and realistic perspective. Make gradual, long-lasting dietary and lifestyle modifications that promote general health and well-being your top priority rather than concentrating on fast cures. You may minimize the hazards involved with quick weight reduction solutions while still achieving durable results by using a balanced approach to weight loss. Recall that long-term habits and behaviors rather than short cuts or extreme measures are what lead to actual health and wellness.

Comprehending Weight Loss Rates

Setting reasonable goals and attaining long-lasting outcomes on your weight reduction journey require an understanding of weight loss rates. Individual characteristics like metabolism, beginning weight, body composition, genetics, age, gender, and general health can all have a substantial impact on weight reduction rates. While some people may lose weight quickly at first, others may develop at a slower rate. In order to comprehend weight reduction rates, keep the following important points in mind:

First Fast Weight reduction: When starting a weight reduction program, it's normal to lose weight quickly this is known as the "honeymoon phase." The main causes of this first weight loss are the loss of water weight, glycogen storage, and smaller food volume in the digestive tract. Although this quick weight reduction can be encouraging, it's crucial to understand that it could not be indicative of long-term fat loss.

Healthy Rate of Weight Loss: One to two pounds per week is typically thought to be a healthy rate of weight loss. This tempo minimizes the risk of muscle loss, nutrient shortages, and metabolic slowing while enabling steady, progressive improvement. A slower rate of weight loss also raises the possibility of long-term weight maintenance.

Elements Affecting Rates of Weight Loss:

Metabolism: People who have greater metabolic rates tend to burn calories faster and lose weight more quickly.

Beginning Weight: Due to higher calorie expenditure, people who are considerably overweight or obese may initially lose weight more quickly.

Body Composition: Since muscle mass has a major impact on metabolism, people who have more muscle mass may lose weight more quickly than people with lower muscle mass.

Gender: Men often lose weight more quickly than women, especially in the early phases of weight loss, due to their higher metabolic rates.

Age: As people age, their metabolism slows down, which may cause older folks to lose weight more slowly.

Genetics: Genetic variables can affect how quickly weight is lost by affecting metabolism, body composition, and how the body reacts to food and activity changes.

Health problems: A person's metabolism and rate of weight loss may be impacted by specific medical problems or drugs.

Plateaus and Stalls: As you get closer to your target weight, it's normal to go through phases of plateauing or slower development. Increased muscle mass, modifications in energy expenditure, or metabolic adjustments can all lead to plateaus. It's critical to have patience at plateaus and evaluate your strategy, adjusting as necessary to keep moving forward.

Non-Scale Victories: Although weight is one indicator of progress, it's equally important to acknowledge and acknowledge non-scale victories like gains in mood, energy, fitness, fit, and general well-being. These progress markers might have equal significance to weight fluctuations and serve as inspiration to stick with your objectives.

Knowing weight loss rates enables you to create a sustainable plan and reasonable expectations for reaching your desired weight reduction outcomes. Be patient with your development and concentrate on making long-lasting, incremental adjustments to your lifestyle, nutrition, and level of physical exercise. You can get long-term weight loss and enhance your general quality of life by placing a high priority on your health and wellbeing.

Evaluating Your Pursuit of Weight Loss

One of the most important steps in figuring out how quickly you can actually lose weight is evaluating your weight reduction objectives. Staying motivated and on track with your weight reduction journey requires setting realistic and doable goals. When evaluating your weight loss objectives, keep the following important aspects in mind:

Assessing your present weight, body composition, and general health status should be the first step. Take into account variables that could affect your weight loss journey, such as your waist circumference, body mass index (BMI), and any current medical concerns. Speaking with a healthcare expert might offer insightful advice catered to your specific requirements.

Desired Weight Loss: Based on your starting point and general health goals, decide how much weight you want to lose and set reasonable expectations. Although it's normal to desire to lose weight rapidly, the secret to long-term success is to aim for sustained weight loss that happens gradually. It is generally accepted that aiming for 1-2 pounds a week is safe and doable for the majority of people.

Timeframe: Evaluate whether your allotted time to reach your weight loss objectives corresponds with a reasonable rate of weight loss. Remember that long-term, sustainable weight loss takes time, patience, and consistency. Don't establish unrealistic deadlines that, if not met, could cause you to get frustrated or disappointed.

Lifestyle Factors: Assess your present way of living, taking into account your eating patterns, degree of physical exercise, stress levels, sleep patterns, and daily schedule. Determine what good changes you can do to support your weight loss objectives. Some examples include adding more fruits and vegetables to your diet, getting more exercise, or giving stress relief and self-care greater importance.

Motivation and Commitment: Consider how committed and motivated you are to changing your lifestyle in order to lose weight. Think about what inspires you to reach your objectives and how you may maintain your motivation and attention while traveling. Establishing SMART goals specific, measurable, realistic, relevant, and time-bound can support sustained motivation and efficient progress monitoring.

Health and Well-Being: Put your health and well-being ahead of the scale's number. In addition to losing weight, concentrate on raising general health indicators including blood pressure, cholesterol, blood sugar, and fitness levels. Recall that maintaining healthy behaviors is the cornerstone of long-term success, and losing weight is only one part of living a healthy lifestyle.

Flexibility and Adaptability: Recognize that progress may not always follow a straight path and maintain your flexibility and adaptability in your approach to weight loss. Be willing to modify your plans, tactics, and deadlines in response to your body's feedback and evaluations of your progress. Keep your commitment to your long-term health and well-being and acknowledge your little accomplishments along the way.

You may create a realistic plan for reaching sustainable weight loss at a speed that suits your unique requirements and preferences by carefully evaluating your weight loss objectives and taking these important elements into account. Keep in mind that development is a journey, and every step you take no matter how tiny brings you one step closer to your objectives. Remember to be persistent, patient, and to put your health and wellbeing first.

Making a Loss of Calories

No matter how soon you want to reach your goals, the first step in reducing weight is creating a calorie deficit. When your body uses less calories than it takes in, you have a calorie deficit, which eventually causes weight loss. To efficiently build a calorie deficit, follow these steps:

Determine Your Basal Metabolic Rate (BMR): The amount of calories required by your body to sustain essential physiological processes when at rest is known as your BMR. Your BMR can be calculated using a variety of online calculators depending on your age, gender, height, weight, and amount of activity.

Calculate Your Total Daily Energy Expenditure (TDEE): This is the total amount of calories you burn during the day, including exercise and physical activity. To estimate your TDEE, multiply your BMR by an activity component, which typically ranges from sedentary to very active.

Establish Your Calorie Intake Goal: Deduct a manageable amount of calories from your TDEE in order to establish a calorie deficit. For a safe and sustainable weight loss of one to two pounds per week, aim for a daily caloric deficit of 500 to 1,000. Steer clear of severe calorie restriction since this can cause metabolic slowdown and nutrient deficits.

Track Your Food Intake: Keep tabs on your daily caloric intake and track your food intake using a food journal, smartphone app, or internet resource. Be mindful of serving sizes, selection of foods, and calories concealed in dressings, sauces, and drinks. To make sure you're remaining inside your calorie target, be truthful and precise in your tracking.

Select Nutrient-Dense Foods: Pay attention to eating foods high in nutrients that are low in calories and high in vitamins, minerals, and macronutrients.

CHAPTER TWO

To promote general health and wellbeing, give priority to fruits, vegetables, lean meats, whole grains, and healthy fats.

Practice Portion Control: To prevent overindulging and maintain your calorie target, pay attention to portion sizes. To help you determine the right portion sizes, use food scales, measuring cups, or visual clues; this is especially important for foods high in calories, such as cereals, nuts, and oils.

Incorporate Protein into Your Meals: Protein is necessary for metabolism, muscle growth, and satiety. To help you feel full and satisfied throughout weight loss, aim to eat lean protein sources like chicken, fish, tofu, lentils, and dairy in each meal.

Keep Yourself Hydrated: To maintain general health and stay hydrated, sip lots of water throughout the day. There are instances when people confuse thirst for hunger, which results in overindulging in calories. To curb hunger and avoid overindulging, try to have water with and in between meals.

Be Aware of Liquid Calories: Sugary drinks, alcoholic beverages, and calorically dense coffee drinks can all contain liquid calories that might lead to weight gain without satisfying your hunger. Choose calorie-free drinks to stay hydrated without consuming additional calories, such as sparkling water, herbal tea, or water.

Combine Diet and Exercise: Although dieting alone can help create a calorie deficit that aids in weight loss, regular exercise can also help to improve overall health and results. To increase muscle mass, boost metabolism, and burn calories, combine cardiovascular, strength, and flexibility training.

To achieve long-term success, keep in mind that establishing a calorie deficit needs to be done in a sustainable and balanced way. Rather than concentrating just on short fixes or drastic measures, try adopting small, long-lasting improvements to your food and lifestyle that support health and well-being. You can safely and successfully lose weight by adhering to a calorie-controlled eating plan on a regular basis and maintaining an active lifestyle.

Including Exercise

Incorporating physical activity is crucial to effectively and efficiently losing weight. Exercise increases metabolism, improves mood and well-being, and helps burn calories. It also improves general health. The following are some methods for including exercise in your weight loss plans:

Choose Pleasurable Activities: Opt for enjoyable physical pursuits that you eagerly anticipate engaging in. Whether it's jogging, walking, cycling, dancing, swimming, or sports, engaging in fun activities improves the probability that you will continue with them over time.

Establish Achievable and Realistic Goals: When setting goals for your physical exercise, consider your preferences, schedule, and current fitness level. As you advance, progressively raise the intensity, duration, and frequency of your goals from manageable starting points.

Make Consistency a Priority: Plan regular workouts throughout the week to achieve consistency in your fitness regimen. Regular exercise maximizes calorie expenditure over time, helps form a habit, and develops momentum. Exercise, even brief exercise sessions, can build up and aid in weight loss.

Incorporate Variety: To target different muscle groups, minimize boredom, and prevent overuse problems, mix up your exercise regimen with a range of activities. To make your workouts engaging and difficult, use functional motions, weight training, and aerobic activities.

Emphasis on Cardiovascular Exercise: Exercises that burn calories and aid in weight loss include jogging, cycling, swimming, and brisk walking. According to health guidelines, try to get at least 150 minutes a week of moderate-intensity or 75 minutes of vigorous-intensity cardiac exercise.

Strength Training: To increase lean muscle mass, speed up metabolism, and enhance body composition, include strength training activities in your regimen. To strengthen and extend your muscles and target your main muscle groups, try using bodyweight workouts, resistance bands, or free weights.

Interval Training: To optimize calorie burning and cardiovascular fitness, include interval training, such as high-intensity interval training (HIIT), in your exercises. Elevating metabolism and burning more calories in less time can be achieved by alternating between periods of high-intensity activity and active rest.

Keep Moving Throughout the Day: Seek chances to add extra movement to your daily schedule to raise your activity levels. To burn extra calories throughout the day, choose for walking or biking instead of driving, stand up and stretch frequently, take the stairs instead of the elevator, and take part in vigorous hobbies or housework.

Listen to Your Body: Pay attention to the cues your body gives you and modify the time and intensity of your workouts accordingly. To avoid overtraining and injury, consider rest and recuperation while pushing yourself to the maximum.

Track Your Progress: To stay motivated and to keep an eye on your efforts, keep track of your physical activity and progress over time. To log exercises, track steps, measure distance, and establish progress targets, use a fitness tracker, diary, or smartphone app.

Including regular exercise in your routine is crucial to losing weight and preserving your general health and wellbeing. You can efficiently increase calorie expenditure, improve fitness, and reach your weight loss objectives by finding activities you enjoy, setting reasonable goals, remaining consistent, and implementing a variety of workouts. Never forget to get medical advice before beginning a new fitness regimen, particularly if you have any underlying medical issues or concerns.

Giving Nutrient-Dense Foods Priority

Making nutrient-dense foods a priority will help you lose weight quickly and effectively while still giving your body the nutrition it needs for general health and wellbeing. Foods high in nutrients are low in calories and high in fiber, vitamins, minerals, and other healthful ingredients, which makes them the perfect option for anyone trying to lose weight. To assist with your weight loss efforts, consider giving nutrient-dense foods top priority.

Emphasis on Whole Foods: Create a diet centered on naturally nutrient-rich whole, minimally processed foods. Fruits, vegetables, whole grains, lean meats, nuts, seeds, and legumes are all included in this. These foods give you vital nutrients and satisfy your hunger while lowering your calorie intake.

Eat a Wide Variety of Colorful Fruits and Vegetables: Packed with fiber, vitamins, minerals, and antioxidants, colorful fruits and vegetables should make up a large portion of your meal. To guarantee that your diet has a wide spectrum of nutrients, try to consume a diversity of colors and varieties. Throughout the day, include fruits and vegetables in meals and snacks to boost nutrition and volume without adding unnecessary calories.

Select Lean Proteins: Make sure your meals contain lean protein sources such beans, fish, shellfish, chicken, tofu, and tempeh. Protein improves muscle repair and maintenance, increases feelings of fullness and satiety, and lowers hunger and speeds up metabolism to help with weight reduction. For maximum support in your weight loss endeavors, try to incorporate protein into every meal and snack.

Select Whole Grains: Refined grains should be avoided in favor of whole grains including quinoa, brown rice, oats, barley, farro, and whole wheat pasta and bread. Whole grains offer longer-lasting energy, help suppress appetite, and balance blood sugar levels. They also contain higher quantities of fiber, vitamins, and minerals. Replace processed grains with whole grains for a boost in nutrient intake and assistance with weight loss during meals and snacks.

Add Good Fats: Include foods high in avocados, nuts, seeds, olive oil, and fatty fish in your diet. These are some sources of healthy fats. Good fats aid in the promotion of sensations of fullness and pleasure and are crucial for hormone production, heart health, and brain function. Even though lipids have a higher calorie content, adding modest amounts of healthy fats to meals can improve flavor and satiety without raising the overall caloric intake.

Reduce Your Consumption of Processed Foods and Added Sugars: Reduce your intake of foods and drinks that are heavy in unhealthy fats, refined carbs, and added sugars because they are empty calories that might cause weight gain. Processed foods, which might undermine weight loss attempts, include sugary snacks, desserts, sugary drinks, fried foods, and packaged snacks. They also frequently lack important nutrients. Whenever feasible, aim for complete, nutrient-dense foods rather than processed ones.

Keep Yourself Hydrated: To maintain general health and stay hydrated, sip lots of water throughout the day. Water helps control hunger and stop overeating. It is also necessary for digestion, metabolism, and cellular function. There are instances when people confuse thirst for hunger, which results in overindulging in calories. In order to stay hydrated and aid in weight loss, try to drink water both before and after meals.

Practice Portion Control: To prevent overindulging and maintain your calorie target, pay attention to portion sizes. To help you determine the right portion sizes, use food scales, measuring cups, or visual clues; this is especially important for foods high in calories, such as cereals, nuts, and oils. In addition to preventing overeating and promoting weight loss, mindful eating and paying attention to hunger and fullness cues can help.

You can support your weight loss objectives while making sure your body gets the nutrients it needs for optimal health and well-being by giving nutrient-dense meals first priority in your diet. Reduce your intake of processed and high-calorie foods and increase your intake of a range of whole foods, such as fruits, vegetables, whole grains, lean proteins, and healthy fats. Recall that the three main components of a healthy diet are moderation, variety, and balance. You need also make durable dietary modifications if you want to successfully lose weight over the long run.

Drinking Water and Losing Weight

Drinking enough water is important for both general health and weight loss. Maintaining enough hydration supports a number of body processes and can aid in weight loss in a number of ways. The following explains how hydration affects weight loss and offers advice on how to drink enough water while trying to lose weight:

Regulating Appetite: Consuming water prior to meals can aid in calorie restriction and appetite control. According to studies, drinking water before meals can make you feel more full, which reduces the amount of calories you eat during the meal. Furthermore, maintaining water helps avoid dehydration, which can occasionally be confused for hunger and result in overindulging in calories.

Increased Calorie Expenditure: Research has demonstrated that drinking water can momentarily raise energy expenditure, also known as calorie expenditure, through a process known as thermogenesis. As the body struggles to bring the water to body temperature after consumption, there is an increase in calories used. Even if the benefit of burning calories is minimal, any amount can help with overall weight loss attempts.

Optimal Metabolism: Your body uses metabolism to turn food and liquids into energy. To maintain optimal metabolism, you must drink enough of water. Dehydration can slow down metabolism, which can make it harder to burn calories and possibly impede weight loss attempts. Maintaining proper hydration promotes healthy metabolism and keeps your body functioning at its best.

Enhanced Exercise Performance: Drinking enough water is essential for both optimum exercise output and recuperation. Your body loses water while you exercise, and being dehydrated increases your risk of weariness and injury as well as performance issues and decreased endurance. Maintaining your fluid intake before, during, and after exercise will help you burn as many calories as possible while working out and maintain your energy levels.

Water Retention and Bloating: Getting adequate water will help minimize bloating and water retention, which can occasionally be linked to changes in body weight. Your body may retain more water when it is dehydrated, which can cause bloating and temporary weight gain. Maintaining hydration can help control fluid balance and reduce water retention, which will result in a more accurate and consistent portrayal of your actual weight.

Suggestions for Including Hydration in Your Dietary Plan:

Drink Water Frequently: Develop the habit of drinking water throughout the day. Aim for 8 to 10 glasses each day, or more if the weather is hot or you're physically active. To stay hydrated when on the run and to sip water in between meals and snacks, always carry a reusable water bottle.

Make Water-Rich Foods a Priority: Include foods high in water, like fruits and vegetables, in your diet. These meals not only help you stay hydrated but also offer important minerals and fiber. Due to their high water content, foods including lettuce, cucumbers, oranges, strawberries, and watermelon can help you meet your daily fluid requirements.

Water Before Meals: Having a glass of water before meals will help curb hunger and cut down on calories consumed. By adopting this modest practice, you can support your weight loss goals by feeling fuller and more content with lesser servings.

Monitor Urine Color: One easy way to check your level of hydration is to observe the color of your pee. Dark yellow urine may suggest dehydration, whereas light or pale yellow pee usually indicates enough hydration. The ideal urine color to indicate adequate hydration is pale yellow.

Drink water before, during, and after exercise to stay hydrated and promote the best possible performance and recuperation. Drink plenty of water while working out, especially in warm or muggy weather, to replenish fluids lost through perspiration.

Restrict Sugary Beverages: Restrict your intake of sugary drinks, which can contribute to excess calories and impede your attempts to lose weight. These include soda, sweetened teas, energy drinks, and fruit juices. For healthy hydration options, go for unsweetened beverages, herbal tea, sparkling water, or water.

As part of any weight reduction plan, making sure you drink plenty of water will help you burn calories, improve your metabolism, promote overall health, and perform better during exercise. To optimize the advantages of hydration for weight reduction and general well-being, incorporate these suggestions for staying hydrated into your daily routine. Regardless of your objectives for losing weight, keep in mind that staying well hydrated is crucial for your health.

Tracking Development

Tracking your weight loss journey and maintaining your motivation and accountability to your goals depend on keeping an eye on your progress. Here are a few successful methods for keeping an eye on development:

Frequent Weigh-Ins: To monitor variations in body weight over time, weigh yourself on a frequent basis without becoming compulsive. Try to weigh yourself once a week, ideally under the same settings (e.g., in the morning before eating or drinking, after using the restroom) and at the same time of day. Maintain a weight log in a diary or on a smartphone app to see patterns and trends over time.

Measurements: Take measurements of your waist, hips, chest, arms, and thighs in addition to your own weight. To measure circumference and monitor changes in inches or centimeters, use a measuring tape. Measurement alterations can sometimes reveal changes in body composition, such as differences in muscle mass relative to fat mass, that are not always evident on the scale.

Body Composition Analysis: To evaluate changes in body composition, take into consideration employing techniques such bioelectrical impedance analysis (BIA) or body fat percentage assessments. These techniques give you a more complete image of your body composition by differentiating between fat and lean body mass (muscle, bones, and organs).

Progress Photos: To visibly track changes in your body's structure and look over time, take progress photos at regular intervals (e.g., once a month or every few weeks). Put on tight clothes or a bathing suit, hold the same posture and angle, and snap comparison shots with your front, side, and back views. Pictures of your progress might serve as a visual reminder of your efforts and an inspiration to keep going.

Fitness Assessments: Monitor parameters including cardiovascular endurance, strength, flexibility, and exercise intensity to gauge your current level of fitness and potential for improvement. To keep track of your workouts, including their time, intensity, and exercises completed, utilize a fitness journal or an app. Establish benchmarks and review your fitness objectives on a regular basis to push yourself and track your improvement.

Dietary tracking: Use a smartphone app or a food journal to record your daily caloric intake, along with information on portion sizes, macronutrient breakdowns, and calorie intake. You may measure your nutrient consumption, find areas for improvement in your eating habits, and make sure you're sticking to your calorie reduction objectives by keeping an eye on your eating habits.

Energy Levels and Well-Being: Throughout your weight loss journey, be mindful of your physical, mental, and emotional well-being. Take note of any changes in your overall well-being, energy levels, mood, digestion, and sleep quality as markers of improvement. More than just the numbers on the scale, your efforts are paying off if you're feeling more cheerful, self-assured, and energized.

Track your adherence to good habits and behaviors that are linked to weight loss, such as consistent exercise, a balanced diet, staying hydrated, and managing stress. To stay on track with your goals, monitor your compliance with your weight loss plan, spot any obstacles or difficulties, and modify your strategy as necessary.

You may properly track your weight reduction journey, maintain your motivation, and make well-informed adjustments to your method as necessary by putting these progress monitoring strategies into practice. Keep in mind that there might not always be a straight road to advancement; there might also be ups and downs. As you work toward reaching your intended weight reduction outcomes, remember to enjoy minor accomplishments, stay focused on your long-term goals, and have patience with yourself.

Overcoming Obstacles and Plateaus

Overcoming obstacles and plateaus is a typical aspect of the weight reduction process, but you may keep moving forward and overcome obstacles if you have the correct techniques and mindset. The following practical advice can help you get past obstacles and plateaus in your weight loss journey:

Examine Your Habits: Pay particular attention to your food, workout regimen, and general way of life to spot any areas where you might have become comfortable or fallen back into old routines.

CHAPTER THREE

Are you eating and burning the same number of calories each day? Do you prioritize self-care, manage stress, get enough sleep, and drink enough water? Evaluating your routines might assist in identifying problem areas and redirecting your efforts.

Change Up Your Workouts: If your fitness regimen has reached a standstill, consider introducing new challenges to your body. To keep your workouts interesting and productive, mix up your routines by incorporating different workouts, adjusting the length and intensity of your exercises, or trying out new classes or activities. In addition to preventing boredom, cross-training can also prevent overuse injuries.

Modify Your Calorie Intake: It's important to frequently reevaluate your calorie intake because your body's needs for calories may alter as you lose weight. Try cutting back on your caloric intake a little bit if you've reached a plateau in order to start losing weight by creating a calorie deficit. Take care not to severely cut calories as this can cause vitamin deficits and slow down metabolism.

Put Quality Sleep First: Since sleep is essential for controlling hormone levels, metabolism, and hunger, make sure you get plenty of it every night. To optimize rest and recuperation, aim for 7-9 hours of excellent sleep each night and create a regular sleep routine. Weight loss can be more difficult when sleep deprivation interferes with hunger hormones and increases desires for unhealthy meals.

Effectively Manage Stress: Prolonged stress can impede weight reduction by inducing hormonal imbalances, emotional eating, and cravings. To increase resilience to stress and encourage relaxation, incorporate stress-reduction strategies into your daily routine, such as yoga, deep breathing exercises, mindfulness meditation, or regular relaxation activities.

Keep Yourself Hydrated: Make sure you drink enough water throughout the day because occasionally, dehydration can pass for hunger and cause overindulgence in food. Regular water consumption might help regulate hunger and minimize weight changes caused by dehydration, particularly before meals.

Practice Mindful Eating: To avoid overeating and to increase awareness of hunger and fullness cues, pay attention to your eating habits and engage in mindful eating. During meals, take your time, enjoy every bite, and concentrate on the whole sensory experience. Steer clear of distractions like screens and multitasking during meals since they might result in calorie overconsumption and thoughtless eating.

Seek Support and Accountability: In trying times, turn to friends, family, or a support group for inspiration, accountability, and words of encouragement. A strong support system may offer direction, compassion, and encouragement to maintain your weight loss objectives.

Be Patient and Persistent: Keep in mind that losing weight is a journey with ups and downs, and that hitting a plateau is common. Remain persistent in your healthy habits, have patience, and have faith that your hard work and persistence will finally pay off. Appreciate your non-scale successes and concentrate on the constructive adjustments you've made to enhance your overall health and wellbeing.

You can overcome obstacles and setbacks in your weight loss journey and keep moving forward in the direction of your intended results by putting these methods into practice and being dedicated to your objectives. Recall that long-term success in sustainable weight loss requires perseverance and determination, but you can overcome setbacks and succeed in the long run.

Possible Hazards of Quick Weight Loss

Although losing weight quickly could sound alluring, there are a number of hazards involved as well as possible harm to your health. The following are some possible dangers connected to losing weight quickly:

Nutrient Deficiencies: Excessive calorie restriction commonly associated with rapid weight loss programs results in insufficient consumption of some nutrients. Deficits in vital vitamins, minerals, and other nutrients that are required for general health and wellbeing may arise from this. Deficits in some nutrients can affect energy levels, immune system performance, and bone health, as well as raise the risk of various health issues.

Muscle reduction: Rapid weight reduction, particularly when coupled with an extreme exercise regimen or a low-protein diet, can result in a significant loss of muscle in addition to fat. Loss of muscle can raise the risk of injury, affect strength and endurance, and impact metabolism. Long-term weight management and maintaining metabolic rate depend on preserving muscle mass.

Reduced Metabolism: The pace at which your body uses calories for energy is known as metabolism, and it can be slowed down by severely limiting your calorie intake. This metabolic slowdown makes it more difficult to lose weight and simpler to gain it back in the future when the body adjusts to preserve energy in response to a drop in calorie intake.

Electrolyte Imbalance: Sudden weight loss, especially when combined with severe calorie restriction or dehydration, can throw off the body's electrolyte balance. Electrolytes, which include sodium, potassium, and magnesium, are vital for maintaining fluid balance, contracting muscles, and neuronal activity. Electrolyte imbalances can cause symptoms like weakness, exhaustion, and lightheadedness, as well as more serious issues like irregular heartbeat.

Gallstones: Quick weight loss may raise your chance of getting gallstones, particularly if it's combined with a low-calorie diet or sudden changes to your body's composition. Solid particles called gallstones develop in the gallbladder as a result of bile component abnormalities. Quick weight loss can alter the makeup of the bile and reduce the amount of time the gallbladder empties, which increases the risk of gallstone development.

Reduced Bone Density: Rapid weight loss can have a detrimental effect on bone health and raise the risk of osteoporosis and fractures, especially when accompanied with insufficient calcium and vitamin D intake. During times of fast weight loss, the body may mobilize calcium from bones to sustain vital activities, which may result in a decrease in bone density.

Gastrointestinal Problems: Constipation, diarrhea, bloating, and discomfort are gastrointestinal problems that can result from abrupt dietary changes, particularly abrupt increases or decreases in fiber consumption. These digestive issues can impair general wellbeing and interfere with regular bowel function.

Mental and Emotional Health: Fast weight reduction diets can have a negative impact on one's mental and emotional well-being, resulting in emotions such as guilt, frustration, and deprivation. Emotional eating, binge eating, compulsive thoughts about food and body image, and other disordered eating behaviors may all be exacerbated by restrictive eating practices. These psychological problems can have a detrimental effect on quality of life and jeopardize long-term weight loss progress.

Yo-Yo Dieting: Yo-yo dieting is the term for the pattern of weight loss and gain that can occur from rapid weight loss programs that frequently provide unsustainable outcomes. Yo-yo dieting can have detrimental consequences on body composition, metabolism, and general health. It can also raise the risk of chronic diseases and make it more difficult to reach and stay at a healthy weight over the long run.

Prioritizing safe, steady weight loss through healthy lifestyle adjustments such as stress reduction, regular exercise, healthy eating, enough sleep, and general self-care is crucial. Before beginning any weight loss program, speaking with a medical professional, registered dietitian, or licensed nutritionist can assist ensure that your strategy is safe, efficient, and customized to your unique needs and health goals. Keep in mind that physical, mental, and emotional wellness are all parts of true health and well-being, which go beyond the number on the scale.

Long-Term Weight Loss Techniques

Prioritizing weight loss techniques that support sustainability, long-term success, and general well-being is essential. Using sustainable weight loss techniques guarantees that you can reach and keep a healthy weight over time, even though quick weight loss may seem enticing. Consider the following long-term weight loss techniques:

Set Achievable and Realistic Goals: Set attainable weight loss targets that put your health and wellbeing before hasty decisions or extreme tactics. It is healthy and sustainable to lose 1-2 pounds of weight gradually each week. Rather than concentrating on achieving quick fixes, try to make long-term lifestyle adjustments.

Emphasis on Whole, Nutrient-Dense Foods: Make fruits, vegetables, lean proteins, whole grains, nuts, seeds, and legumes the main components of your diet. These foods are also very fiber- and nutrient-dense. These meals assist you in reaching and maintaining a healthy weight while offering vital nutrients, encouraging fullness, and supporting general health.

Practice Portion Control: Pay attention to the amounts you consume and follow your body's signals of hunger and fullness to prevent overindulging. Aim to fill half of your plate with fruits and vegetables, one-quarter with lean protein, and one-quarter with whole grains or starchy vegetables. Use smaller plates, bowls, and utensils to help reduce portion sizes.

Keep Yourself Hydrated: To maintain general health and wellbeing and to stay hydrated, sip lots of water throughout the day. There are instances when people confuse thirst for hunger, which results in overindulging in calories. To curb hunger and avoid overindulging, try to have water with and in between meals.

Include Physical Activity: Include physical activities that you enjoy in your routine, such as cycling, swimming, walking, jogging, or dancing. Aim for two or more days of muscle-strengthening activities each week in addition to at least 150 minutes of moderate-intensity or 75 minutes of vigorous-intensity aerobic activity per week.

Make Sleep and Stress Management a Priority: Get the recommended amount of sleep each night (7-9 hours for adults), and make stress-reduction methods like yoga, deep breathing exercises, mindfulness meditation, or regular relaxation techniques a priority. Weight loss might become more difficult when hormones that control hunger and desires for unhealthy foods are disturbed by long-term stress and sleep deprivation.

Practice Mindful Eating: To avoid overeating and to increase awareness of hunger and fullness cues, pay attention to your eating habits and engage in mindful eating. Eat mindfully of your surroundings, take your time, and enjoy every bite. Steer clear of distractions like screens and multitasking during meals since they might result in calorie overconsumption and thoughtless eating.

Seek Accountability and Support: Encircle yourself with people who can provide accountability, inspiration, and encouragement, such as friends, family, or a weight loss support group. Having a support network can help you stay motivated, empathetic, and on track with your weight loss objectives, particularly when things are tough.

Be Patient and Persistent: Keep in mind that it may not always be easy to lose weight sustainably, and that it requires time and work. Remain persistent in your healthy habits, have patience, and have faith that your hard work and persistence will finally pay off. Appreciate your non-scale successes and concentrate on the constructive adjustments you've made to enhance your overall health and wellbeing.

You can attain and retain a healthy weight over time while promoting general health and well-being by giving sustainable weight loss techniques top priority and implementing small, long-lasting adjustments to your food, exercise routine, and lifestyle choices. Recall that consistency is the key to long-term success and that every little step toward living a better lifestyle matters.

Summary

In summary, each person's road towards weight loss is unique and varies greatly. Even though it's normal to want to lose weight quickly, it's important to approach weight loss with an emphasis on long-term sustainability, general health, and well-being.

Crash diets and other drastic methods of weight loss can be dangerous and have detrimental effects on one's physical and mental well-being. To achieve and maintain a healthy weight over time, it is essential to employ sustainable weight loss strategies that place a high priority on stress management, balanced eating, regular exercise, enough sleep, and self-care in general.

You can achieve sustainable weight loss results that support your overall health and well-being by setting reasonable goals, concentrating on whole, nutrient-dense foods, practicing portion control, staying hydrated, adding physical activity, putting sleep and stress management first, engaging in mindful eating, asking for help and accountability, being patient and persistent, and following through on your goals.

Keep in mind that physical, mental, and emotional wellness are all parts of true health and well-being, which go beyond the number on the scale. Accept the weight-loss journey as a chance for constructive lifestyle adjustments and personal development, and acknowledge each little accomplishment as it occurs. You may thrive in all facets of life and reach your weight loss goals with commitment, consistency, and long-term health in mind.

THE END